I0422396

The Science, Techniques and Tips for How To Get To Sleep

written by

Debbie Brewer

Cover Artwork by

Eloku

Copyright © 2019 Debbie Brewer

First published in November 2019 by
Lulu.com

Distributed by Lulu.com

All rights reserved. No part of this
book may be reproduced by any
mechanical, photographic, or
electronic process, or in the form of a
phonographic recording. Nor may it be
stored in a retrieval system ,
transmitted or otherwise be copied for
public or private use, other than for
fair use as brief quotations embodied
in articles and reviews, without prior
written permission of the author.

ISBN-13: 978-0-244-22575-9

First Edition

The author of this book does not dispense medical advice or prescribe the use of any technique as a form of treatment for physical, emotional or medical problems. The intent of the author is only to offer information of a general nature to help you in your search for emotional and spiritual well-being. In the event you use any of the information in this book for yourself, the author assumes no responsibility for your actions.

Contents

Foreword

As a former staff nurse, I am acutely aware of the need to sleep and the difficulties we sometimes face when trying to get to sleep.

My former job meant that I had to work shifts, including night shifts, which made falling into a regular sleeping routine difficult. It also meant I had to find a way to be able to achieve adequate sleep in the daytime to be able to continue to work safely at night, and then be able to revert back to sleeping at night at the end of my night shifts. I can only liken it to being jet lagged, all of the time.

Similarly, it is not only shift workers who may struggle with getting off to sleep and then staying asleep long enough to be able to wake up in the morning feeling refreshed and ready for the day. We all have times during our lives when sleep has eluded us for varying reasons.

I have therefore researched in depth the many things we can do to make getting to sleep and staying asleep easier, and have written this self-help book to share my findings. After all, without enough sleep, our day to day lives can become severely affected.

With so many tried and tested ideas, you are most certainly going to find a method that works for you here. So get reading, try out these techniques, and then sleep well!

Why We Need To Sleep

Sleep allows us to process the day's information, and restore and strengthen our bodies. But scientists can still not tell us exactly how or why this happens. However, it is apparent that it is absolutely vital for health and well-being.

Our bodies appear to be pre-programed to slumber for several hours each night, during which time we become unconscious and paralysed. When you consider this, it does seem a bizarre behaviour, but one which is essential to properly maintain.

When we achieve a 'good night's sleep', we wake up in the morning feeling refreshed and ready for the day. And this in turn gives us a 'feel good' reaction, which can enhance and set the mood for the rest of the day. Similarly, lack of sleep can induce a fatigue and sluggishness that can stay with you for the entire day, and that is something we all want to avoid. Especially when it affects your ability to work, or interact with friends and family.

Achieving sufficient sleep makes our brain and body function correctly. It helps repair and restore our organs, tissues and muscles, strengthen our immune systems and synthesize hormones. In daytime, new experiences cause the brain to build new connections. When we are sleep, those connections are prioritised in order of importance. The important ones are strengthened and the unimportant ones are discarded. Waste information is cleared away, so the brain becomes uncluttered. The ability to prioritise and interact is improved after proper sleep and ideas and plans become clearer.

Poor sleep negatively affects learning, memory retention, mood and emotions. When we are sleep deprived but awake, some parts of our brain can become inactive, even though we are still awake, leading us to have the feeling of being 'slow witted', sluggish or 'half asleep'.

Poor sleep in the long term may lead to:

- A strain on family relationships.
- A struggle to maintain a social life.
- Finding it hard to complete everyday tasks.

- Feel hungrier, snack more and put on weight as a result.
- Being unable to feel refreshed when getting up.
- Feeling of unwarranted exhaustion during the day.

Notably, children need more sleep than adults, as they are learning at a much faster rate, learning essential skills for life such as language, social and motor skills. Hence the brain needs more time in sleep mode to process what the child has learnt while awake.

Types Of Sleep

Scientists have identified four main stages of sleep that we go through during the night. Each stage has a significant purpose that makes them important. These are:

- Stage One: Drowsy Light Sleep
- Stage Two: Light Sleep
- Stage Three: Deep Sleep
- Stage Four: REM (Rapid Eye Movement). This is when dreaming occurs.

These stages typically progress from stage one through to stage four in order, with each stage lasting between 5 to 15 minutes. As the night continues, the REM stage can become longer, even up to an hour towards the end of the night. The complete cycle takes an average of 90 to 110 minutes, and then begins again at stage one.

We also have brief moments of wakefulness during the night, of which we are generally unaware, and these usually it occur at the end of stage four before the cycle restarts at stage one again.

The Stages of Sleep

Stage One

Stage one of sleep is a drowsy light sleep. During this stage, the brain produces alpha and theta waves. There may be slow eye movements, and you can be easily aroused and woken. Muscle tone relaxes, and at this stage some people experience 'hypnic jerks', which are sudden involuntary harmless muscle spasms. These jerking movements can be severe enough to wake you up. Taking a brief 'catnap' would be classed as resting in stage one of sleep.

Stage Two

Stage two is a light sleep, where slow eye movements may still occur, but you are not aroused or woken quite so easily. The brain produces short sudden bursts of faster brain waves called sleep spindles. Your body temperature will decrease slightly and your heart rate will slow. If you were to 'power nap' you would want to wake up after this stage of sleep.

Stage Three

Stage three is a deep sleep. The brain produces slower waves called delta waves. It can be difficult to wake someone from a deep sleep. Sleep talking, sleep walking and night terrors are most likely to happen during this stage. During this sleep period, the body secretes growth hormone. The body repairs and regenerates tissues, bone and muscle, and strengthens the immune system. The heart is slow and regular and the muscles are very relaxed. You rarely dream during this stage and there is no eye movement.

Stage Four

Stage four is when REM (rapid eye movement) sleep occurs. The eyes will move around quickly. You can be woken more easily from this stage, but may feel groggy as a result. This stage is when dreaming occurs as the brain is more active, but the muscles are effectively paralysed so the body is inactive. Heart rate and blood pressure increase and breathing can become faster, irregular and shallow.

During REM sleep, emotion, learning and memory are regulated as the brain is consolidating and processing information from the previous day and clearing away things that are not needed.

Stages of Sleep

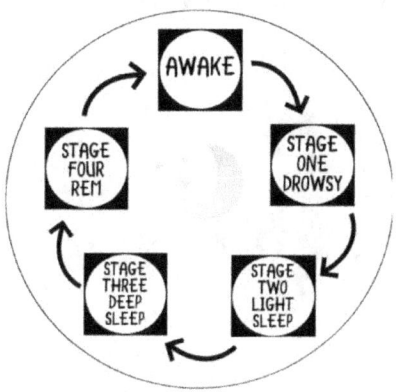

The full cycle takes between 90 – 110 minutes and then begins again.

Time Spent In Each Sleep Stage During One Night

(Based on average values)

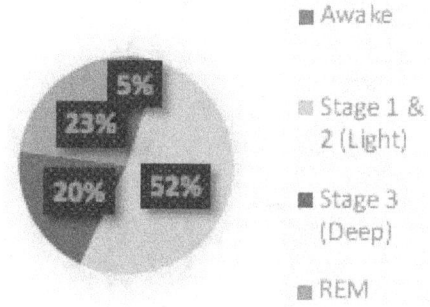

Summary:

Awake: 5%

Stage 1 & 2 (Drowsy & Light Sleep): 52%

Stage 3 (Deep Sleep): 20%

Stage 4 (REM): 23%

Brain Activity During Sleep

During each stage of sleep, our brain activity differs, and when measured, the brain produces different brain waves. As we go through the stages of sleep, the brain waves get longer as our brain activity decreases. But as you enter the REM stage, the brain activity increases again because you are dreaming.

Brainwave Activity During Sleep

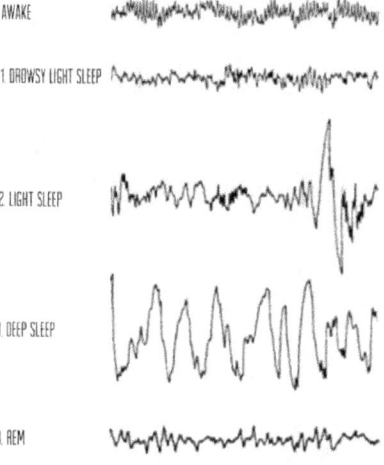

How Long Should We Sleep?

As individuals, we all have different requirements for sleep, based on our lifestyles. Having a job that entails a lot of physical activity may mean you need more sleep to recover. Looking after young children, or getting a good exercise routine, and many other physical factors may have the same effect.

Having certain chronic conditions may also leave you tired and in need of more sleep. Some conditions may have the opposite effect and cause you to sleep less.

Similarly, our genetic makeup may also dictate whether we need more or less sleep than the next person. We are each unique in our requirements.

Hence, exactly how many hours sleep we need is impossible to accurately predict. Instead we have to take an average and offer a range of results.

The following chart displays average figures, which when analysed, basically show that the older we get, the less sleep we need and the less stage three deep sleep we require.

We will discuss more about the implications of age and sleep in a later chapter.

How Long We Sleep

(based on average sleep hours)

Age	Hours
New Born	12 - 18
3 months – 1 year	14 - 15
1 – 3 years	12 – 14
3 – 5 years	11 – 13
5 – 12 years	10 – 11
12 – 18 years	8.5 – 10
18 – 25 years	7.5 – 9
26 – 64 years	7 – 9
65 + years	7 – 8

Data taken from Hafco Ltd, (2018)

How Long We Spend in Deep Sleep

(Based on average values)

Age	Deep Sleep Hours
New Born	2.4 – 3.6
3 months – 1 year	2.8 – 3
1 – 3 years	2.4 – 2.8
3 – 5 years	2.2 – 2.6
5 – 12 years	2 – 2.2
12 – 18 years	1.7 – 2
18 – 25 years	1.5 – 1.8
26 – 64 years	no data
65 + years	no data

Data taken from Hafco Ltd, (2018)

Why Do We Have Trouble Sleeping?

Medical Conditions

Many medical conditions can affect getting to sleep, staying asleep, and attaining sufficient sleep to be able to maintain your normal daily activities. Below are listed a few of them.

As with all medical worries, should you feel you are affected by any of the following, then you should seek advice and assistance from a medical practitioner / doctor.

Acid Reflux / Heartburn

Lying down will often make heartburn more severe, causing discomfort which will keep you awake. Avoiding heavy and fatty foods, coffee and alcohol will help. Sleeping with the upper part of the body elevated will also help. Finally, you may talk to your doctor regarding medication to supress the heartburn.

Anxiety

Persistent excessive anxiety, worry and apprehension will cause problems with falling asleep and staying asleep.

Depression

People with clinical depression are very likely to experience difficulty getting to sleep, fitful sleep and early awakening.

Mental Health Disorders

Bipolar disorder is often associated with sleep disruption, often not being able to sleep over a period of several days (manic) before 'crashing' and staying in bed for a long period (depressive).

During an episode of schizophrenia, a person may sleep very little. Between episodes, their sleep may improve, but will rarely be a 'normal' amount of deep sleep.

Cardiovascular Disease / Heart Failure

Heart failure may lead to wakefulness caused by shortness of breath. Elevating the upper part of the body may help.

Hyperthyroidism

An overactive thyroid gland will produce too much thyroxine, which, among other things, stimulates the nervous system, making it hard to settle to sleep, and causing night sweats.

Diabetes

If the blood sugar levels are not well controlled in a person with diabetes, then among other symptoms, they may experience night sweats, a frequent need to urinate, and hypoglycaemia (low blood sugar crisis). Also, if nerves in the legs are damaged due to diabetes, then involuntary night time movements and pain may occur.

Musculoskeletal Disorders

Pain and swelling associated with arthritis can make falling asleep and staying asleep difficult as pain can occur when trying to change sleeping positions overnight.

Painful ligaments and tendons associated with fibromyalgia are also likely to affect sleep

Kidney Disease

People with damage to their kidneys can have a build-up of waste products in the blood that may cause insomnia or restless legs syndrome.

Neurological Disorders

Dementias such as Alzheimer's Disease may disrupt a person's ability to regulate sleep as they may become unaware of the time of day and the 'body clock' malfunctions.

People with epilepsy can be prone to insomnia and tend to attain less REM sleep. Night time seizures are also a problem, and are experienced by one in four people with epilepsy.

Parkinson's Disease will likely cause people to suffer from insomnia and fitful sleep, often disturbed by involuntary tremors and movements.

Respiratory Disorders

Asthma, emphysema, bronchitis and other respiratory conditions may also cause sleeping difficulties due to shortness of breath or coughing.

If you suspect you have any underlying medical issue which could be the cause of your sleep problems, then contact your doctor for medical advice and help.

Other Things That Can Affect Sleep:

Stress

Medication

Pregnancy

Menopause

Weight

Age

Drug abuse

Alcohol, caffeine, nicotine

ADHD

Noise

Uncomfortable beds

Jet lag

Shift work

A room that's too hot or too cold

Young children and babies

Pets

And more.

Insomnia

Insomnia occurs when you regularly have problems sleeping. It is an habitual sleeplessness or an habitual inability to sleep. Chronic insomnia is disrupted sleep that occurs at least three nights per week and lasts for at least three months.

You may have insomnia if you regularly experience the following over a space of months or even years:

- Find it hard to go to sleep
- Lie awake at night
- Wake up several times during the night
- Wake up early and cannot get back to sleep
- Still feel tired after waking up

- Find it hard to nap during the day even though you feel tired
- Feel tired and irritable during the day
- Find it difficult to concentrate during the day because you feel tired.

You can check your 'sleep score' using the following test adapted from the Sleepio self help program:

Sleep Score Test

Question One

Thinking about a typical night in the last month, how long does it take you to fall asleep?

- 0-15 minutes:
  score 4 points
- 16-30 minutes:
  score 3 points
- 31-45 minutes:
  score 2 points
- 46-60 minutes:
  score 1 point
- More than 61 minutes:
  score 0 points

Question Two

Thinking about a typical night in the last month, if you wake up, how long are you awake for in total?

- 0-15 minutes
    score 4 points
- 16-30 minutes
    score 3 points
- 31-45 minutes
    score 2 points
- 46-60 minutes
    score 1 point
- More than 61 minutes
    score 0 points

Question Three

Thinking about the last month, how many nights a week do you have a problem with your sleep?

- 0-1 nights
    score 4 points
- 2 nights
    score 3 points
- 3 nights
    score 2 points
- 4 nights
    score 1 point
- 5-7 nights
    score 0 points

Question Four

Thinking about a typical night in the last month, how would you rate your sleep quality?

- Very good
  score 4 points
- Good
  score 3 points
- Average
  score 2 points
- Poor
  score 1 point
- Very Poor
  score 0 points

Question Five

Thinking about the past month, to what extent has poor sleep affected your mood, energy, or relationships?

- Not at all
    - score 4 points
- A little
    - score 3 points
- Somewhat
    - score 2 points
- Much
    - score 1 point
- Very much
    - score 0 points

Question Six

Thinking about the past month, to what extent has poor sleep affected your concentration, productivity, or ability to stay awake?

- Not at all
    - score 4 points
- A little
    - score 3 points
- Somewhat
    - score 2 points
- Much
    - score 1 point
- Very much
    - score 0 points

Question Seven

Thinking about the past month, to what extent has poor sleep troubled you in general?

- Not at all

    score 4 points
- A little

    score 3 points
- Somewhat

    score 2 points
- Much

    score 1 point
- Very much

    score 0 points

Question Eight

How long have you had a problem with your sleep?

- I don't have a problem (or I've had a problem for less than one month)
    score 4 points
- 1-2 months
    score 3 points
- 3-6 months
    score 2 points
- 7-12 months
    score 1 point
- Longer than a year
    score 0 points

Results

The lower your 'sleep score' result, the higher the chance that you may be suffering from insomnia.

If you scored 0 – 15 points, then your sleep score is poor and this would suggest that you are experiencing a number of symptoms of insomnia.

If you scored 16 – 24 points, then your sleep score is ok, but you have indicated that you experience a few symptoms of insomnia.

If you scored 25-32 points, then your sleep score is good to excellent, which suggests that you are not experiencing insomnia at the present time.

If you think you are suffering from chronic insomnia, then consider getting help and advice from your local medical practitioner / doctor.

Sleep And Aging

Trends in sleep change as we get older. Babies can spend up to 50% of their sleep in the REM stage, whereas adults will usually spend only 20% of their sleep in REM.

As we get older, we find it harder to get to sleep and stay asleep. We wake up more often and we spend more time in the lighter stages of sleep than the deeper ones, especially the REM stage. Older people, on average, wake up three or four times each night, and are more likely to be aware of their wakeful times.

Older people are also more likely to suffer from conditions that wake them in the night, such as nocturia, (the need to get up and urinate), anxiety, pain and discomfort from chronic conditions, menopause, etc. They are also more likely to suffer from insomnia, sleep apnea and severe snoring, restless leg syndrome, narcolepsy, and hypersomnia (excessive daytime drowsiness).

Older people are more likely to feel a level of fatigue during the day due to lack of sleep. They are also more likely to start to feel tired and sleepy earlier in the evening and wake earlier in the morning, unlike young people who will be more wakeful until late in the night and more tired in the morning. This is due to our altering circadian rhythms, which control the timings of our body functions, including that of sleep.

Body Weight And Sleep

There is research to suggest that sleep directly affects weight loss. Researchers at the Kaiser Permanente Center For Health Research in Portland, US, in 2011, carried out sleep and stress trials on 472 obese adults.

They found that "chronic stress may trigger hormonal reactions that result in an intake of energy-dense foods, so that eating becomes a "coping behaviour" and palatable food becomes "addictive". Lack of sleep may also affect hormones associated with feelings of fullness or hunger." These hormones are ghrelin and leptin.

They concluded that people who slept well, for between six and eight hours were more likely to be able to lose weight than those who slept less or more. Also, people affected by stress were less likely to sleep well, making their level of motivation for sticking to weight loss programmes more difficult.

Researchers at John Hopkins University School Of Medicine, in the US, also did sleep trials with 77 overweight participants. After six months of exercise and weight loss dieting, the researchers found that belly fat was reduced on average by 15% and sleep time and quality improved.

It is thought that being overweight increases the chances of developing obstructive sleep apnea, where the airway can become temporarily, partially or completely blocked, leading to sudden and frequent wakening during the night.

Overall, it is apparent that being overweight can cause sleep disturbances. Similarly, lack of sleep can cause weight gain. Hunger and appetite appears to increase and we are more likely to load up on calorie dense foods and carbohydrates. And the fatigue caused by lack of sleep causes reduced motivation and energy levels, leading to less physical exercise, in turn, leading to weight gain.

This all seems like a vicious circle! If you are overweight, the only thing to do is break the circle. Partake in weight loss diet and exercise, even if you don't feel like it due to lack of sleep. Eventually you will find that you will sleep better. Then you will find it easier to lose weight.

Your motivation will increase and the vicious circle will reverse, this time in your favour.

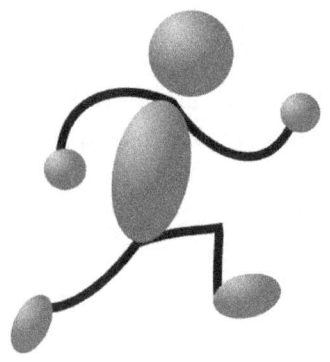

Vicious Circle of Sleep and Weight

Vicious circle relationship between exercise and poor quality sleep:

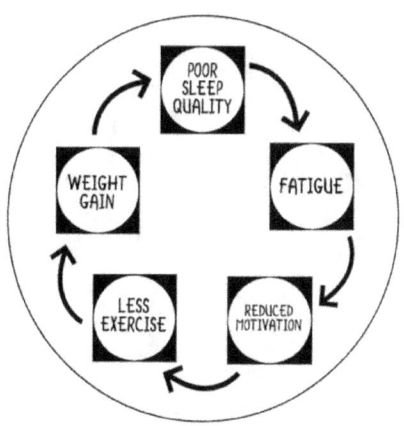

Vicious circle relationship between food and poor quality sleep:

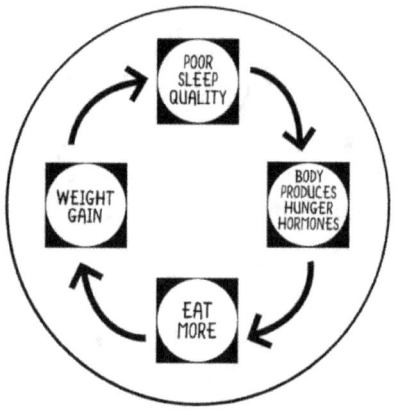

Vicious circle relationship between exercise and good quality sleep:

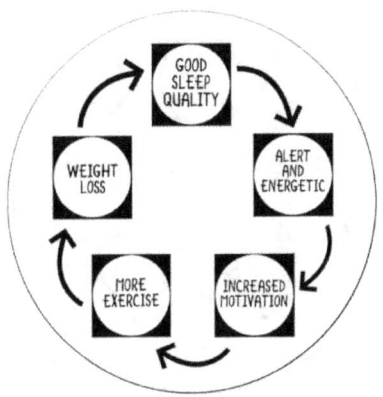

Vicious circle relationship between food and good quality sleep:

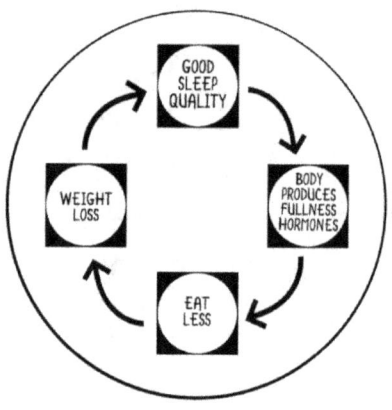

Sleep Differences Between Men And Women

According to the National Sleep Foundation, (2019), research has shown that there are notable differences between men and women with regards to sleep.

The hypothalamus in the brain controls our circadian rhythms, which in turn have an effect on our body clocks. The circadian rhythms between men and women differ.

Men

The circadian cycles of men tend to run slightly longer than the twenty four hour clock, meaning they are slightly longer than women's by an average of six minutes.

Men tend to feel less tired in the evening. They are more likely to be 'night owls'.

Men find it harder to recover from periods of sleep deprivation.

The risk of heart problems related to lack of sleep is lower in men.

Men spend more time in the REM stage of sleep than women, meaning that they dream more.

Women

The circadian cycles of women tend to run slightly shorter than the twenty four hour clock, meaning they are slightly shorter than men's by an average of six minutes.

Women tend to wake earlier in the morning. They are more likely to be 'early birds'.

Women are more susceptible to insomnia.

Women are more likely to suffer from restless leg syndrome.

Women are more likely to have a dip in energy at night time when doing night shift work.

Women are better at catching up on sleep after a shortfall.

Women spend more time in the deep sleep stage than men.

Menstrual cycles, pregnancy and menopause make it harder for women to sleep.

Women tend to require up to twenty minutes more sleep in a night than men.

Does Dreaming Affect Sleep?

Dreams can occur in any stage of sleep, but most usually and most vividly in the REM stage.

As yet, scientists do not conclusively understand why or how we dream.

The psychologist, Sigmund Freud (1856 – 1939) believed that dreams were a window into our subconscious, revealing a person's:

- unconscious desires
- thoughts
- motivations.

Modern experts believe that dreams are a way for our brains to process and clarify our thoughts and emotions of the day. They can also help solve problems and incorporate memories.

In one experiment, researchers conducting dream studies, woke their subjects up just as they were drifting into REM sleep. By depriving them of the dream phase of their sleep, they found that these subjects experienced:

- increased tension
- anxiety
- depression
- difficulty concentrating
- lack of coordination
- weight gain
- increased tendency to hallucinate.

According to the National Sleep Foundation, (2019), on average, people over the age of 10 years old dream between 4 to 6 six times every night, (a total of up to two hours each night), during the REM stage, but we tend to forget between 95-99% of our dreams the next morning. Children under the age of ten years old, tend to dream for only 20% of the time they are in the REM stage.

Being a normal part of sleep, dreams do not normally affect the quality of sleep. Usually we forget the dream as we wake and become unaware that we were dreaming.

However, there are times when they will affect sleep. For example, after waking from a nightmare, it may be difficult to get back to sleep. And if it was particularly lucid, it may stay with you, making your mood low for the rest of the day. This is referred to as a 'bad-dream hangover'.

The difference between pleasant dreams and bad dreams does not seem to affect the length of time in each stage of sleep, although it has been suggested that it is more difficult to switch between the REM and non-REM stages after a bad dream.

Temperature

While asleep, the natural body temperature drops by 1 – 2 degrees.

Body temperature fluctuations during the day and night

Temp (centigrade)

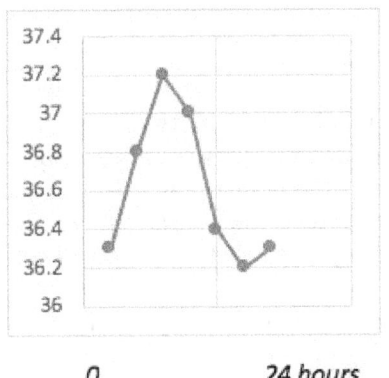

Keeping cool at night will aid sleep.

Sleeping In Hot Weather

Trying to get to sleep, and stay asleep during periods of hot weather can be a challenge. But there are things you can do to make it more comfortable for yourself and help you settle.

Use air conditioning units if available to cool the environment.

Use one or more fans to keep the air moving.

Use breathable cotton bed sheets for comfort.

Wear breathable nightclothes or sleep naked.

Consider using specific 'cooling' sheets made typically from bamboo or organic cotton.

Freeze a gel filled eye mask to use at night.

Put sheets into a plastic bag and stow in the freezer. Then place them on the bed just before bedtime.

Fill a sock with rice and freeze it, then place it on your pulse points.

Turn off all plug sockets, as they will emit a small amount of heat.

Keep curtains and blinds closed in the daytime to prevent the room from overheating from sunlight.

Freeze water in a hot water bottle for use in the bed.

Open windows to aid air flow.

Since heat rises, put the mattress on the floor, or sleep downstairs.

Remove excess blankets.

Spritz the sheet with cool water.

Spritz your face with cool water.

Put ice in a dish and place in front of a fan. This will create a cool breeze around the room.

Use cooling aloe gel on your skin.

Apply cold compresses to neck, wrists, insides of elbows, around the groin, behind the knees and around ankles.

Sleep alone. Sleeping with a partner will double the body heat in the room.

Keep all doors in the house open to encourage circulation of air.

Take a cool shower or bath before bed to cool the body

Hang a wet sheet over an open window to encourage a cool breeze.

Drink a small cool glass of water before bedtime, and keep a glass of water by your bedside to consume during the night.

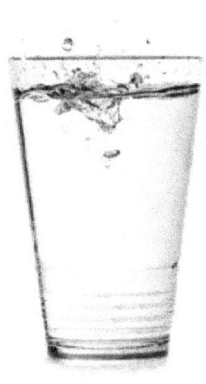

Only eat light dinners, no heavy foods.

Use a buckwheat or foam pillow which will tend to keep your head cooler.

Soak your feet in cold water just before bedtime.

Napping

To nap means to sleep lightly or briefly, especially during the day. To take a nap means to take a short sleep. It can be a wonderful way to refresh yourself during the day, but a nap should be done wisely. Taking the wrong kind of nap can have a significant effect on your night time sleeping habits.

According to a report by Pew Research (2009) a third of US adults nap each day.

The benefits of napping include:

- Boosts brain function
- Increases focus, concentration and accuracy
- Improves critical thinking skills

- Lowers stress
- Enhances creativity
- Improves memory
- Increases levels of tolerance
- Lifts mood
- Enhances learning ability
- Improves energy levels and physical performance

Some businesses, such as Google, Uber, Zappos and Ben & Jerrys, have become so aware of the benefits of a nap, that they've installed dedicated nap areas in their headquarters, believing that their employees will become more efficient as a result.

There are several different types of naps:

The Catnap (or 'forty winks')

This is a brief nap where you are resting in stage one of sleep only, usually only lasting approximately ten minutes. For just a small amount of time, this type of nap can feel very recuperative, and you will experience cognitive improvement, particularly if you are sleep deprived from the night before.

The Power Nap (or Coffee Nap / Nap a Latte)

The power nap is a longer nap, whereby you aim to wake up after stage two of the sleep cycle, after around 20-25 minutes of sleep. It is also referred to as the Coffee Nap (or more trendily, the Nap a Latte), because of a neat little trick: If you drink a cup of coffee just before you take this nap, then set your alarm for twenty minutes, when you wake up, the caffeine will be just starting to kick in, so you will feel refreshed and alert.

The Nasa Nap

According to a study by Nasa in 1995, the most effective nap for peak performance and alertness lasts 26 minutes.

In a study on sleepy military pilots and astronauts, they also found that napping for 40 minutes improved performance by 34% and alertness by 100%. This 40 minutes nap time is referred to as the Nasa Nap.

The Bad Nap (The Slow-Wave Sleep Nap)

Waking after a nap lasting between 30-60 minutes, can leave you feeling groggy as you are waking from a deep slow wave sleep stage. However, once the grogginess passes, (which usually takes another 30 minutes) you will experience the same amount of cognitive improvement as that of a catnap. Hence, this nap apparently has no real benefit over a ten minute nap.

The Full Sleep Cycle Nap (or Refresher Nap)

This nap should last at least 90 minutes, and will encompass the full sleep cycle, including the REM stage. It will enable you to wake up feeling fully rejuvenated.

Naps can be taken as either a planned habitual nap or as an emergency nap.

For example, it is very common to feel drowsy early in the afternoon, typically around 2pm. Maintaining an habitual power nap around this time can improve your performance at work or home.

Taking an emergency unplanned nap can be very beneficial when you know you have to complete a specific task and want to be in your best cognitive and physical form to do it. For example, if you are driving for a long period on the motorway, you may experience fatigue. Pulling over at a service station and taking an impromptu nap before you continue will allow you to safely go on with your journey.

The most important point to napping, is that it should not affect or impair your night time sleeping pattern. Choosing the right type of nap for you, depending on its purpose, will enable you to maximise you efficiency and help feel good about yourself for the rest of the day, and still attain a good night's sleep.

Comfort And Sleep Position

Sleeping in comfortable surroundings is essential for a good night's sleep. Being uncomfortable in bed can cause getting to sleep difficult, and waking several times in the night and then again in the morning with stiff aching joints, especially back and neck pain.

The National Sleep Foundation (2019) found that on average, 41% of people in the United States preferred to sleep in the foetal position while only 8% preferred to sleep on their back.

People fall into one of three categories of sleeping positions: Side, back and stomach. Each position has its pros and cons.

Sleeping On Your Side

There are three variations of side sleeper positions:

- Log position (with straightened arms and legs)
- Foetal position (with bent arms and legs)
- Yearner position (straight legs and arms extended outwards)

As a side sleeper, provided that you are sleeping on an even surface, the spine should remain in a natural alignment in these positions.

The advantages of sleeping on your side include:

- Better air circulation through the breathing passages

- Less pressure on the heart
- Less likelihood of heartburn
- Less painful for people with hip pain and scoliosis

The disadvantages of sleeping on your side include:

- Restricted blood flow in the shoulders and arms
- More pressure on the stomach and lungs

The ideal mattress type for someone who sleeps on their side would be firm enough to support the body without allowing it to sink.

Sleeping On Your Back

There are three variations of back sleeper positions:

- Soldier position (straight arms, one leg bent, one leg straight)
- Starfish position (both arms extend over the head and both legs slightly bent at the knee)
- Savasana position (arms and legs are straight)

As a back sleeper, the spine will maintain a natural alignment.

Sleeping on your back means that you are less likely to suffer with acid reflux, but you are, however, more likely to suffer with sleep apnea and snoring.

The ideal mattress for someone sleeping on their back would be a medium to firm one, that provides even support from head to toe, but soft enough for the lumbar region to be supported.

Sleeping On Your Stomach

Sleeping on your stomach is a position called Freefall. One or both arms can rest beneath the pillow and the legs are fully extended and slightly apart.

The spine is not in natural alignment as the mass of the stomach causes you to sink too deeply into the middle of the mattress.

Sleeping on your front does reduce the likelihood of sleep apnea and snoring, but studies have shown that sleeping in this position does lead to tossing and turning, which can lead to sleep disruption.

If you sleep on your front, you should choose a mattress that is firm enough to support you and stop you from sinking down in the middle.

Choosing A Pillow

Choosing the right pillow and mattress is essential.

- If you sleep on your back, then a thinner pillow, with extra filling in the lower third will cradle your neck.
- If you sleep on your side, then a firmer, thicker pillow is needed to fill the gap between the ear and shoulder.

- If you sleep on your stomach, then you need a very thin pillow.

The thickness of a pillow is called it's loft. There are three levels of loft; low, medium and high.

Pillows with low loft:

- Are less than 3 inches thick
- Are good for small head sizes
- Are good if your weight is over 230 lbs
- Are good if your shoulders are narrow

Pillows with medium loft:

- Are 3 – 5 inches thick

- Are good for average head sizes
- Are good if your weight is between 130-230 lbs
- Are good if you have average shoulder width

Pillows with high loft:

- Are more than 5 inches thick
- Are good for large head sizes
- Are good if your weight is over 230 lbs
- Are good if you have broad shoulders

Back Pain Sleeping Position

If you suffer with an achy back, adjusting your sleeping position can help.

- Sleeping on your stomach puts extra pressure on your lower back, around the lumbar region, so if you can, try sleeping on your side or your back
- If you sleep on your back, try putting pillows under your knees.
- If you sleep on your side, put a pillow between your knees and pull your knees a little closer to your chest.

Preferred Type Of Mattress (US)

(based on average values in the United States in 2017, data gathered by Statista)

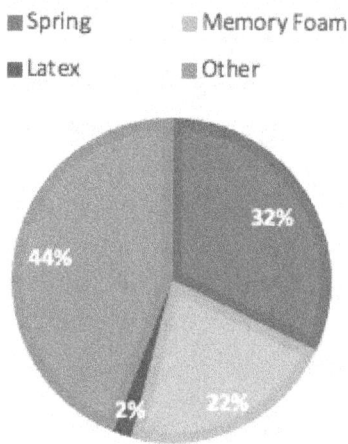

MATTRESS TYPE PREFERENCES

■ Spring   ■ Memory Foam

■ Latex   ■ Other

The most popular type of mattress in the United States in 2017 was the spring mattress, followed by the memory foam mattress.

As well as considering your sleeping position when choosing your mattress, you should also consider your weight.

As a side sleeper:

- if you weigh less than 130 lbs, then you should choose a soft to medium-soft mattress.
- If you weigh 130 – 230 lbs, then you should choose a medium to medium-firm mattress.
- If you weigh over 230 lbs, then you should choose a

medium-firm   to   firm
mattress.

As a back sleeper:

- If you weigh less than 130 lbs, then you should choose a medium-soft to medium mattress.
- If you weigh 130 – 230 lbs, then you should choose a medium to medium-firm mattress.
- If you weigh over 230 lbs, then you should choose a medium-firm   to   firm mattress.

As a stomach sleeper:

- If you weigh less than 130 lbs,   then   you   should

choose a soft to medium-soft mattress.
- If you weigh 130-230 lbs, then you should choose a medium-soft to medium mattress.
- If you weigh over 230 lbs, then you should choose a medium-firm to firm mattress.

When choosing the right pillow and mattress, it is important to get it right to achieve that perfect night's sleep. Do your homework and consider it as an investment in your health.

Bathing

A warm bath or shower at night, as part of your regular night time routine before you go to bed will aid sleep in addition to several other benefits.

Benefits of a warm bath or shower

- Relaxes the muscles
- Lowers body tension
- Helps alleviate headaches and migraines
- Reduces swelling
- Reduces anxiety
- Acts as a nasal decongestant
- Removes toxins from the skin
- Opens pores and cleans the skin

Using aromatherapy oils and salts in your bath can enhance the benefits.

There are also other health-related benefits to be had.

Heart Health

Taking a warm bath will make your heart beat a little faster, giving it a healthy workout. The warmth will make the blood less viscose (thinner), allowing it to flow, improving circulation to your extremities. This can lower blood pressure and improve cardiac function.

Respiratory Health

Immersing your chest in the warm water can improve your lung capacity and the steam can clear your airways and your sinuses. You are able to breathe deeper and slower and so oxygen intake is improved.

Immunity

With increased oxygen intake and improved circulation caused by bathing in warm water, your immunity is naturally boosted.

Digestion

By improving your blood circulation through taking a warm bath, you are naturally helping your digestion. Recent studies have also shown that bathing can have a small effect of reducing blood sugar levels.

Hormones

Taking a warm bath can increase your levels of the hormone, serotonin. This is produced in the brain and is associated with the feeling of happiness and general well-being.

Prescribed medication

Some medications can cause sleep disturbances and insomnia as a side effect. The following list is not exhaustive, and not everyone will experience the same side effects or the same level of severity.

If you have any concerns regarding your medication, then consult with your pharmacist or medical practitioner.

Beta Blockers:

- Insomnia
- night time awakenings
- nightmares

Clondine:

- Disrupted REM sleep
- early morning awakening
- nightmares

Corticosteroids:

- Insomnia
- decreased REM sleep

Diuretics:

- Increased night time trips to the toilet
- calf cramp when asleep

Medication containing alcohol:

- Suppressed REM sleep
- disrupted night time sleep

Medication containing caffeine:

- wakefulness that may last several hours

Nicotine replacement products:

- Insomnia
- disturbing dreams

Sympathomimetic stimulants:

- difficulty falling asleep
- decreased REM sleep
- decreased non-REM deep sleep

Theophylline:

- Wakefulness

Thyroid Hormone:

- Difficulty falling asleep
- fragmented sleep
- insomnia

Medication To Help You Sleep

Being unable to sleep does not mean you should turn to the use of prescribed medication at first. But if you are suffering from chronic insomnia, then it may be worth talking to your doctor for advice.

But beware.

'At best, sleeping pills are a temporary band aid. At worst, they're an addictive crutch that can make insomnia worse in the long run.' (Robinson et al, 2019).

The best use of sleeping pills is on an infrequent, 'as required' basis, to avoid dependency.

Disadvantages Of Taking Sleeping Pills

- They may have side effects.
- You may build up a tolerance to them if taken over a period of time, rendering them less effective.
- You may develop a drug dependence or addiction to them.
- You may experience withdrawal symptoms if you suddenly stop taking them.
- They may interact with other medication you may be taking.
- After a course of sleeping pills, the insomnia may return even worse than before.

- Taking the sleeping pill may mask an underlying problem, ie the real cause of the insomnia.

If you feel that medication may help you resolve your sleep problems, then always talk to your doctor. Should you be prescribed sleeping pills, read the labels and instructions carefully and follow them, and always consult your doctor if you experience any side effects or have any concerns.

% Adults Who Use Medication To Aid Sleep

(based on average figures in the United States in 2010, from the National Center for Health Statistics)

Percentage

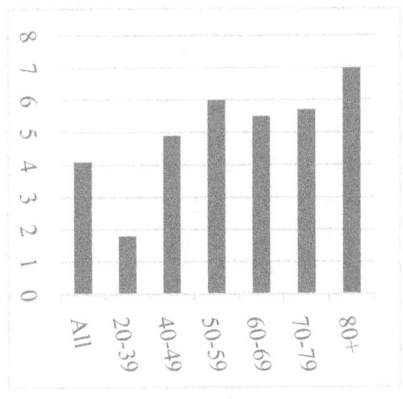

Age range

As you can see from the chart, there is a general trend for older people to use medication to aid sleep, with a substantial increase in their use starting from the age of forty.

This ties in with our previous chapter on how age and sleep are related, where it was shown that older people are more likely to suffer with sleep problems than younger people.

Routines

Getting into a regular routine that you repeat each night before you go to bed is an excellent way of letting the subconscious mind know that it's time to settle down ready for sleeping.

Similarly, partaking in specific activities each day, such as exercise and regular meal times will aid maintaining a healthy sleeping pattern.

When you get ready for bed, maintain routine bathroom habits.

Go to bed at the same time every day.

Get up at the same time every day.

Plan for seven to nine hours of sleep each night. As you get into a sleep routine, you will find out how much sleep works for you, but it should be within this range.

Avoid watching TV in bed. It will only provide more stimulation to keep the brain awake.

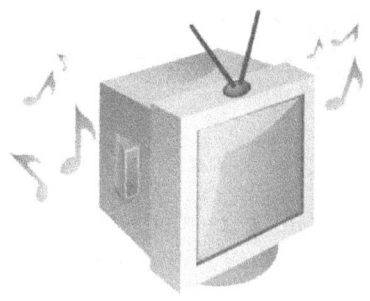

Avoid listening to the radio in bed, unless it is calm gentle relaxing music, playing very quietly. You don't want to hear sounds that stimulate the brain.

Avoid using electronic devices in bed such as laptop, mobile phones or tablets. The blue light they emit will disrupt your ability to settle to sleep. You can often use the settings on a device to switch off the blue light. However, the information you are browsing on the device will be processed by the brain, causing extra brain activity, which you want to minimise before sleeping.

Avoid using social media before sleeping.

Exercise moderately every morning. Morning is the best time to partake in vigorous activity.

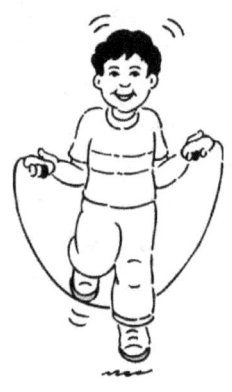

Spend 30-60 minutes doing some kind of relaxing task to 'wind down' before going to bed each evening.

Get into the habit of writing a diary or journal on the day's events, specifically the positive events, before you settle to sleep.

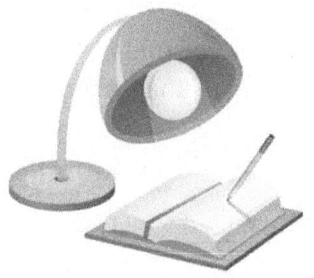

Avoid napping. If you do choose to nap in the daytime, take no more than a twenty minute nap, to avoid reaching the deep sleep part of the sleep cycle. A good way to nap, is to drink a cup of coffee just before you nap. It takes around twenty minutes for the caffeine to kick in, so when you wake up you will be fresh and alert.

Food And Drink

The type and quantity of food that you eat in the evening can dramatically affect your sleeping habits, as can the fluid you drink.

Try to take your meals at a similar time each day, and not too close to bedtime, and regulate the amount that you intake. A heavy meal just before bedtime will leave you feeling uncomfortable and unable to settle to sleep. Too much fluid before bedtime will make you wake up during the night to take extra visits to the toilet.

Avoid eating or drinking heavily close to bedtime.

Avoid a high carb diet.

Avoid sugary foods

Avoid sugary drinks

Avoid excess alcohol.

Avoid nicotine.

Avoid caffeine.

Drink a sleep promoting herbal tea

Eat a small amount of sleep promoting food

Foods That Promote Sleep

Some foods, in small quantities actually promote sleep. Aim to have a small amount of one of the following, a short while before settling to sleep.

Almonds

Turkey

Kiwi Fruit

Tart Cherry juice

Fatty Fish

- Salmon
- Tuna
- Trout
- Mackerel

Walnuts

White rice

Eggs

Bananas

Oatmeal

Cottage cheese

Milk

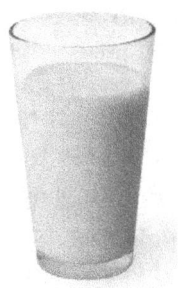

Warm milk is often considered a cosy comforting bedtime drink.

Herbal Teas That Promote Sleep

It is well known that certain types of herbal teas will reduce tension and encourage a sense of calm in the body, as well as provide many other health benefits, making them excellent pre bedtime beverages.

Remember to limit the amount of fluid you use to make the tea. One small cup is ample.

Choose one or a combination of the following herbs to make your herbal tea. Pour boiling water over it and leave to brew for a couple of minutes. Then strain the fluid, allow it to cool, and sip.

You can combine these suggested herbs to make a tea that works best for you to help you reach a state of tranquil relaxation.

Herbal teas also hold many other health benefits. Consider other types of herbal teas and make them a regular part of your daily diet.

Herbs To Choose

Chamomile Tea

Valerian Root Tea

Lavender Tea

Lemon Balm Tea

Passionflower Tea

Magnolia Bark Tea

Mint Tea

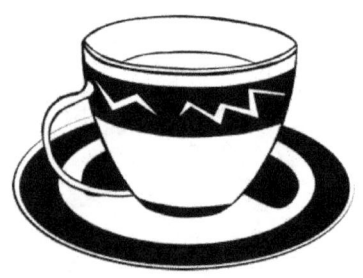

Mind Clearing Mantras

The use of mantras is a type of meditation. The subject of the mantra should be conducive to rest, relaxation and sleep and related to yourself personally.

Choose from a variety of suggested mantras.

Pick a phrase or mantra that has meaning for you, and keep repeating it in your head. Focus carefully on the meanings of the words to stop your thoughts from straying. It will help calm a busy mind and ease you gently into sleep.

For insomnia, choose one of the following mantras:

"I welcome sleep into my being"

"Nothing is left undone"

"I rest inside a pause"

"I make peace with time"

"With each breath, I am closer to sleep"

"I embrace my dreams"

"I am becoming more relaxed with every breath"

"My mind and body are ready for sleep"

"I am calm and still"

"I release this day"

For anxiety, choose one of the following mantras:

"The world is sleeping and all is well"

"I release all worry and celebrate the possibilities"

"Let it be"

"My body is a source of calmness"

"Where I am is where I am meant to be"

"I let go of what I do not need"

"I choose to feel at peace"

"All experiences are helping me grow"

"I have enough, I do enough, I am enough"

"Around me and within me I find stillness"

"Relax, release, rest"

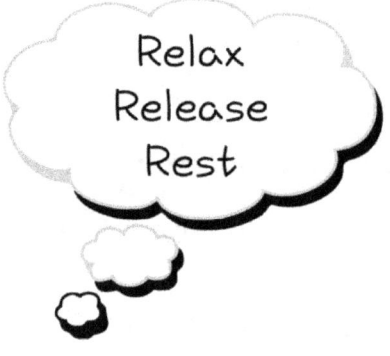

For happiness, choose one of the following mantras:

"I allow myself to be happy"

"I welcome all forms of positivity into my life"

"Each day my life grows more beautiful"

"I am capable"

"I am grateful for this time to rest"

"I am surrounded by love and support"

"I am in complete control of my emotions"

"All I need comes when I need it"

"I love and approve of myself"

"I am comfortable in my own skin"

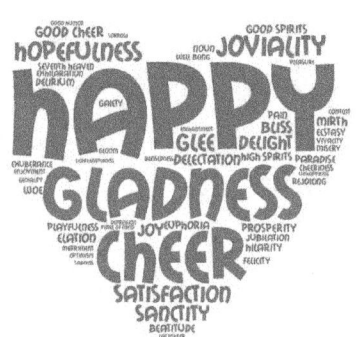

For focus, choose one of the following mantras:

"My mind is calm and my body is relaxed"

"Every heavy thing falls away"

"I am free to be in the present"

"I am, I am, I am"

"I breathe in peace and exhale tension"

"I am here and now"

"I feel every part of me relaxing"

"It is always now"

"I enjoy the feeling of stillness"

"I put my thoughts aside in this moment"

Yoga Meditative Mantras:

"Har Har Mukunday" – "The infinite creator liberates me"

"Ang Sang Waheguru" – "The Infinite Being is within me and

vibrates in ecstasy in every molecule and cell of my being"

"So hum" – "I am that"

"Sa Ta Na Ma" – "Infinity Birth Death Rebirth"

Environment

Creating a calm comfortable environment, conducive to rest and relaxation, is absolutely essential for a good night's sleep.

Lower the room temperature to around 67 - 70°F (20°C). A cooler room will aid sleep. A hot room will make sleeping difficult and uncomfortable.

Make your room dark at night. Use blackout curtains or blinds if necessary. The body is more likely to relax and the brain will rest if the room is darkened.

Minimise artificial lights from devices like alarm clocks. Turn any clocks or devices that emit light away from you. Older clocks that tick might be worth placing in another room if they disturb you.

Ensure you have a comfortable mattress. Upgrade it if necessary. We spend up to a third of our lives in bed, so it is worth investing in a good quality comfortable mattress.

Ensure your pillow is comfortable for the curvature of your neck.

Use a weighted blanket or duvet.

Upgrade your mattress and bedding every 5 – 8 years.

Make sure the linen you have on your bed is fresh and clean and is made from a good quality breathable material such as cotton.

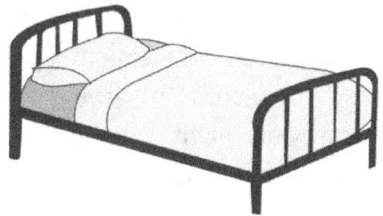

Wear breathable fabric nightclothes to help remain a comfortable temperature while asleep.

Minimise external noise.

Make sure the bedroom is clean and fresh.

Pets

Some people sleep better knowing their cat or dog is sleeping with them on their bed or in their bedroom. It could be the thought of the extra security of having the pet nearby at night, or the cosy warm feeling you get from a pet that snuggles up to sleep with you.

Others will find that the pet may keep them awake or wake them in the night. If this is the case, then consider making your pet sleep in another room.

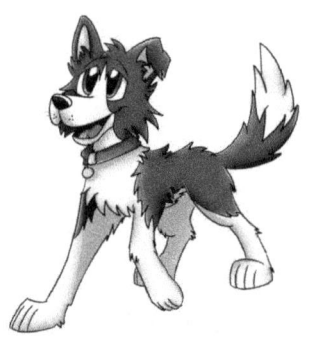

Stress

Stress is a major reason for being unable to get to sleep. When you have had a stressful day, you may find it difficult to stop your brain from going over the events that have caused the stress. Your brain may be playing it over and over in your mind and it can feel impossible to switch it off.

Similarly, long term stress can also cause sleep to be disrupted. When you are going through a stressful period in your life, you may find it difficult to relax, get to sleep, and stay asleep. If this is not addressed, then more serious sleep disorders can emerge.

How to reduce stress before sleep

Most suggestions to remove stress and aid a sense of calm in the body are to be found in other sections within this book as they overlap in other topics, but here are a few extra tips.

Take a warm bath before bed to aid muscle and joint relaxation.

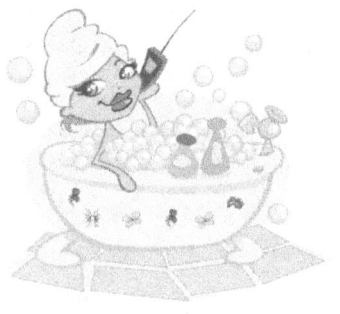

Have a relaxing massage before bed.

Practice slow deep breathing.

Practice Yoga to improve breathing patterns and body movements that release stress and tension.

Practice meditation to enhance melatonin levels and achieve a sleepy state.

Practice mindfulness to focus on the present and remove worries while falling asleep.

Bathe your feet in hot water before bed to aid relaxation.

Sleep Apnea and Snoring

Sleep apnea is a potentially serious sleep disorder, whereby breathing while asleep repeatedly stops and starts. This condition can lead to other complications such as heart problems.

If you think you might suffer from sleep apnea, then you should seek medical advice from a doctor.

There are three kinds of sleep apnea:

Obstructive Sleep Apnea

This occurs when the muscles of the throat relax. It is the most common form of sleep apnea.

Central Sleep Apnea

This happens when the muscles involved in breathing do not receive correct signals, or signals are interrupted from the brain.

Complex Sleep Apnea (Treatment-Emergent Central Sleep Apnea)

This is when a person has a combination of both central and obstructive sleep apnea.

Symptoms of Sleep Apnea

- Snoring; Snoring is very common among people with sleep apnea, though it is possible to have the condition and not snore. Similarly, if you snore, it does not necessarily mean you have sleep apnea.

- Having a partner notice that you tend to have episodes where you stop breathing while asleep.
- Having a partner notice that you have episodes of gasping for air while asleep.
- Frequently waking up with a dry mouth.
- Frequently having a headache in the morning.
- Suffering from insomnia. (Night time wakefulness).
- Suffering from hypersomnia. (daytime sleepiness).
- Poor attention span in the daytime.

- Increased irritability.

Sleep Apnea Remedies

As already said, sleep apnea can lead to increased risk of serious health problems such as:

- heart problems
- high blood pressure
- type 2 diabetes
- metabolic syndrome
- liver problems.

However, certain lifestyle changes can reduce the risks:

- maintain a healthy weight.
- Don't smoke
- Exercise regularly
- Don't drink alcohol excessively.

- Sleep on your side or abdomen.

If natural remedies don't work, your doctor might suggest airway pressure devices such as a CPAP machine (continuous positive airway pressure), or an oral appliance or surgery.

Snoring

Snoring is very common. In the US, it is estimated that nearly 45% people snore.

It is caused when the air passing through your throat as you sleep, causes throat tissue to vibrate.

As already said, you can snore and not have sleep apnea. However, snoring can wake you up.

Also, if your partner snores, this can also lead to you struggling to get to and stay asleep.

Snoring Remedies

- If you are overweight, then lose weight.
- Try altering your sleep position. You are more likely to snore if you lie on your back. Try sleeping on your side or front.
- Elevate the upper half of your body.
- Use nasal strips or external nasal dilators.

- Treat any chronic allergies, such as hay fever or pet allergies, that may restrict air flow through the nose or mouth.
- Reduce your alcohol intake.
- Avoid sedative type medication before bedtime.
- Avoid smoking.
- Keep the bedroom humid
- Use an anti-snore pillow
- Try singing several times a day to strengthen throat muscles.
- Stay well hydrated
- Avoid dairy products
- Avoid fatty and sugary foods late at night.
- Take a warm bath or shower at night.

- Sew a tennis ball into the back of your pyjamas, so that you can't roll onto your back while sleeping.
- Try using peppermint or eucalyptus aromatherapy.
- Use steam inhalation before bedtime.

If your partner keeps you awake by snoring, you might consider sleeping in a different room.

Restless Leg Syndrome (Willis-Ekbom Disease)

Restless leg syndrome is a common long term neurological disorder whereby a person experiences an unpleasant feeling in the legs, such as an aching, tingling or crawling, leading to an irresistible urge to move to alleviate these feelings. However, the action of moving only temporarily relieves the discomfort.

Rarely, it can also occur in other parts of the body.

Symptoms of discomfort can range from mild, to intolerable, and as they usually (though not always) occur at night, they can cause severe sleep disruption.

The symptoms are most likely occur at the early part of the night, when a person is trying to get to sleep, but it can wake them up at any time.

It is estimated that up to 10% people experience this phenomena.

There are two types of restless leg syndrome:

Primary or Idiopathic Rest Leg Syndrome.

This happens gradually, progressively and can get worse with age. It will tend to come and go. It often starts when a person is in their forties, and there is a likely genetic link, but no definite known cause.

Secondary Restless Leg Syndrome.

This happens suddenly, often as a result of another condition, such as nerve problems, pregnancy, iron deficiency and chronic kidney failure.

Restless Leg Syndrome Remedies

There are medications to help treat restless leg syndrome. You should see your doctor for advice.

Other remedies which may help alleviate the symptoms include:

- Soak in a warm bath.

- Massage your leg muscles.
- Apply a heat pack or a cold pack, or even try alternating the two.
- Try stretching.
- Try walking around.
- Try a little yoga
- Try Tai Chi.
- Try acupuncture.
- Try distracting yourself by reading or watching television.
- Exercise regularly during the day.
- Avoid alcohol, especially before bedtime.
- Avoid caffeine, especially before bedtime.
- Establish a regular sleeping routine.

Sleep Promoting Supplements

Many supplements have been found to promote sleep. Some supplements work better for some than others, and you should try to find which work best for you. You could also try a combination of supplements.

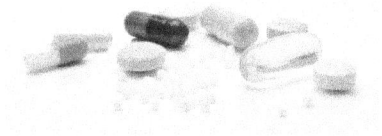

Important: Check with a qualified medical practitioner / doctor if you are on any medication or have any condition which may be affected by taking a specific supplement.

Supplements which are thought to promote sleep

Melatonin

Ginkgo Biloba

Glycine

Valerian Root

Magnesium

L-theanine

Lavender

Tryptophan

Gamma-aminobutyric acid (GABA)

Aromatherapy

The use of aromatherapy has been known to be helpful to aid rest and sleep for hundreds of years.

Aromatherapy scents can be delivered in varying methods. Try using an oil diffuser in your bedroom, or a small bag of dried herbal scents, or an air, or pillow, mist or spray.

Keep the scent light. Do not overuse it. A strong smell be seem pungent and may have the opposite effect of keeping you awake.

Try different scents, and see which ones work for you.

Scents which aid sleep

Lavender

Damask rose

Chamomile

Cedarwood

Vanilla

Valerian Extract

Sandalwood

Juniper

Lemon

Bergamot

Frankincense

Ravensara

Marjoram

Geranium

Rose

Ylang Ylang

Jasmine

Sleep Techniques

There are many sleep techniques to choose from, aside from counting sheep, all of which have shown varying levels of success.

Some are more complicated than others. Some will seem very simple.

Try them out and see which work for you.

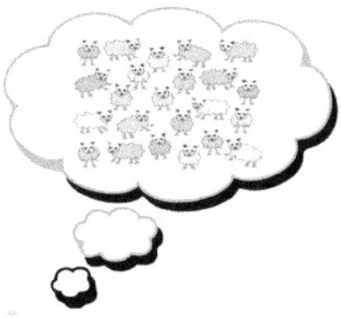

The 4-7-8 Breathing Method

- Place the tip of your tongue behind your upper front teeth.
- Exhale completely through your mouth and make a whoosh sound
- Close your mouth and inhale through your nose while mentally counting to four.
- Hold your breath and mentally count to seven.
- Open your mouth and exhale completely, making a whoosh sound and mentally counting to eight.
- Repeat the cycle.

Paradoxical Intention

Sleep is achieved through deliberately trying to stay awake instead of trying to force yourself to sleep. This may sound absurd, but it can work.

Do something that will deliberately stimulate the brain, such as read a good fiction paperback book or deliberately think about something.

The harder you try to stay awake, the more your brain will feel like it needs to sleep.

Step Breathing Method

- Lie in a comfortable sleeping position and close your eyes.
- Breathing in while counting slowly to four.
- Breathe out counting slowly to four.
- Breathe in counting to four.
- Breathe out counting to five.
- Continue counting four in and five out until you feel you can count six out.
- Continue counting four in and six out until you feel you can count seven out.
- Continue counting four in and seven out until you feel you can count eight out.

- Continue this pattern, so that you eventually you inhale to a count of four and have a long deep exhale.
- You will have slowed your breathing pattern to a pattern conducive to sleeping which can now naturally occur.

Visualisation

Visualise a place that makes you happy, such as sitting on a beach. Picture the environment that makes you feel peaceful and concentrate on good thoughts.

Focus on the details in the image and imagine the sounds, smells and feelings invoked by the image.

Think about what you are doing in this special place. Are you pushing your toes through the warm sand? Is the wind breezing across your face?

Imagine every possible detail of this place, to stop your thoughts from straying.

Free Mind Running

This method takes a little practice and imagination. It is good if you have a busy mind that won't settle and needs distraction.

Lie in a comfortable sleeping position with your eyes closed.

Imagine you are putting on a pair of trainers and lace them up.

Imagine yourself starting to run. In your imagination there are no limits and nothing you cannot do.

Imagine running upstairs, into the loft, through the window, across a roof top, down a ladder, over a fence, through a wood, up a slope, down an alley, up a fire escape, back on the roofs, up a pitched roof, past the chimney,…. Make it up as you go and keep it going.

Continue the run in your mind and if your imagination drifts, then go with it. Let it flow.

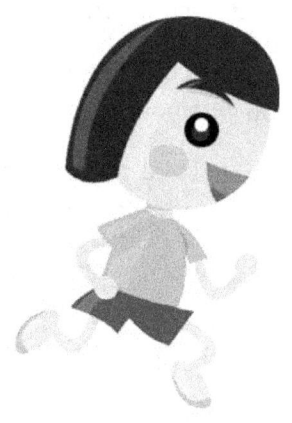

Calm Breathing Method

- Close your eyes.
- Listen carefully to your natural breathing.
- As you inhale slowly, imagine the breath reach and fill each part of your body, right down to your fingers and toes.
- As you slowly exhale, feel all breath and tension leaving your body completely.
- Continue to focus on your breathing and repeat.

Guided Imagery

- Close your eyes and relax.
- Visualize a favourite calm scene.
- Now visualize partaking in an activity within this scene, such as reading a book or dancing etc.
- Concentrate on building this scene in your mind, allowing the story to grow in detail and depth.
- Guide the story as it develops in your imagination.

Progressive Muscle Relaxation

- Lie comfortably on your bed.
- Raise your eyebrows as high as you can, hold for 5 seconds, then relax and breathe deeply for 10 seconds.
- Clench your eyes shut, hold for 5 seconds, then relax and breathe deeply for 10 seconds.
- Open your mouth widely, hold for 5 seconds, then relax and breathe deeply for 10 seconds.
- Raise your shoulders as high as you can, hold for 5 seconds, then relax and breathe deeply for 10 seconds.
- Take a deep breath to tighten your chest, hold for

5 seconds, then relax and breathe deeply for 10 seconds.

- Suck in your stomach, hold for 5 seconds, then relax and breathe deeply for 10 seconds.
- Tighten your right arm muscles and clench your right fists, hold for 5 seconds, then relax and breathe deeply for 10 seconds. Repeat with the left.
- Tighten your buttocks, hold for 5 seconds, then relax and breathe deeply for 10 seconds.
- Tighten your leg muscles and pull your toes upwards, hold for 5 seconds, then relax and breathe deeply for 10

seconds. Repeat with the left.

- Curl your toes downwards, hold for 5 seconds, then relax and breathe deeply for 10 seconds.

Sound Meditation

- Lie comfortably and close your eyes.
- Listen to quiet 'non-threat' sounds, or 'white noise', such as ocean waves or wind breezing through trees or road traffic. (if you want, you can download an app to your phone for these sounds).
- Focus on these sounds and let your mind drift.

Bhramari Pranayama Breathing Exercise

- Close your eyes and breathe deeply in and out.
- Cover your ears with your hands.
- Place each index finger above each eyebrow and cover your eyes with the rest of your fingers.
- Put gentle pressure on the sides of your nose and focus your mind on your brow area.
- With your mouth closed, breathe out slowly and deeply through your nose and hum the 'Om' sound.
- Repeat.

Three Part Breathing Exercise

- Inhale slowly and deeply.
- Exhale slowly and fully while focussing on your body and how it feels.
- Repeat, each time slowing your exhale breath until, it is twice as long as the inhale breath.

Diaphragmatic Breathing Exercise

- Lie on your back and bend your knees over a pillow
- Place one hand flat against your chest and the other on your stomach.
- Breathe slowly through your nose, keeping your chest hand still, so that only the stomach hand rises and falls with each breath.
- Now purse your lips and continue to breathe slowly
- Repeat breathing using your stomach muscles so that your chest doesn't move.

Alternate Nasal Breathing Exercise

- Sit with your legs crossed.
- Place your left hand on your knee and your right thumb against your nose.
- Fully exhale and close the right nostril.
- Inhale fully through your left nostril.
- Release your right nostril and exhale.
- Now repeat on the other side.
- Your breathing will become calm and you will begin to feel sleepy.

Papworth Method

- Sit up in bed.
- Inhale deeply through your mouth and while counting to four.
- Fully exhale through your nose while counting to four.
- Repeat. While breathing, focus on the rise and fall of your stomach.
- When you feel calm and sleepy, try settling down to sleep.

Kapalbhati Breathing Exercise

- Inhale deeply though your nose.
- Purse your lips and exhale three times more slowly than your inhaled.
- Repeat.

Box Breathing

- Fully Exhale.
- Inhale slowly while counting to four.
- Hold your breath and count to four.
- Exhale fully while counting to four.
- Hold again while counting to four.
- Repeat.

Story Telling

Read a paperback book, but make sure its fiction. Non-fiction will not calm the mind.

Alternatively, start your own fictional tale in your mind and imagine a story. Be as detailed as you can and literally see your story playing out in your mind as you imagine it.

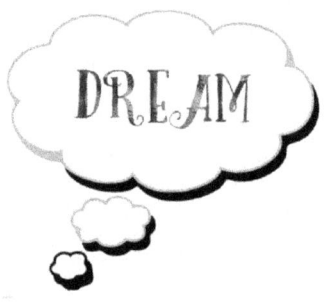

Recall

Mentally recall the day as if it were a story starting with the most recent and working back to the beginning of the morning.

As you remember each event, focus on the detail, the conversations, the sights and sounds and the sensations.

Sleep Ritual

Create a personal sleep ritual that you stick to each time you get ready for bed, so that your subconscious mind recognises that it must calm down and get ready to sleep.

It may be to listen to a certain piece of music, or wash, or read, or even take a gentle walk.

Always maintain the same ritual and ensure it is not mentally stimulating.

Reflective Log of Your Day

Keep a reflective log, where you write down every event of the day, including how each event has made you react and feel.

Use a pen and paper rather than a laptop or smart device.

Toe Curling

This is a simple, yet surprisingly effective method to help you get off to sleep.

- Curl your toes and squeeze them closed.
- Hold for two seconds.
- Release.
- Repeat.

Writing

- Set a timer for 20 minutes.
- With a pen and paper, start freely writing every thought that randomly enters your head.
- Stop when the timer goes off.
- Your brain will feel relieved of thoughts and ready to sleep.

Change The Past

- Take an experience that you feel bad about, eg. A fight with family, a failure at work etc.
- Think carefully over the facts of the event.
- Ask yourself, "What did I learn from this?" "What is good about this?" "How does this make me a stronger or better person?"

Roll Your Eyes

- Close your eyes and become aware of your body and your breathing.
- Roll your eyes down and exhale deeply and slowly.
- Roll your eyes up and inhale deeply and slowly.
- Repeat.

Stretching

- Put your legs up against a wall.
- Stretch your arms above your head.
- Stretch out your back.
- Then relax.

Belly Rub

- Starting at your navel, rub your belly in bigger and bigger circles in a clockwise direction as you inhale deeply.
- As you fully exhale, rub your belly in decreasing circles back to your navel.
- Repeat.

More Helpful Tips

Here are a few more helpful tips that are not covered in the previous sections of this book.

Try plunging your face into cold water. This seems to make the body respond by wanting to rest after the shock of the cold water.

Wear socks so feet are warm and cosy. A cosy feeling will induce a sense of calm.

Use the bathroom just before going to bed to avoid waking in the night.

Keep a notepad nearby and write down any worries before going to sleep so they don't play on your mind.

Write down details you need to remember for the next day, so you don't stay awake worrying about them.

Try humming gently.

If one specific thing is keeping you awake, such as an email that needs to be sent, then do it, and then go back to bed.

If the room is not dark, then try wearing an eye mask.

If there is noise that you cannot avoid, try wearing ear plugs.

Imagine in detail doing a task that you find boring, such as dusting.

Pretend to be tired. Imagine the feelings and sensations of tiredness. The pretence can trick the brain into sleepiness.

Adjust your sleeping position to find the most comfort. If it is hot, then spread out.

Increase bright light exposure during the day, especially sunlight.

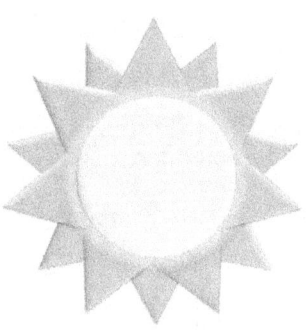

If you can't resist using electronic devices before sleeping, then see if you can block the blue light they emit through their settings, or through using an app, or by wearing blue light blocking glasses.

Note:

If sleep issues are ongoing, then get medical advice from a qualified doctor to rule out a sleep disorder.

End

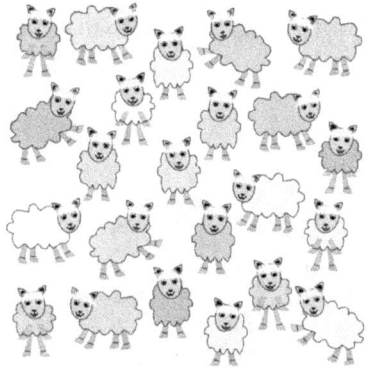

References

Breene, S (2015) 24 Tricks To Survive Hot Summer Nights, www.greatist.com

Brown, N (2015) 18 Charts That Will Help You Sleep Better, www.buzzfeed.com

Elliott, B (2017) The 9 Best Foods To Eat Before Bed, www.healthline.com

Felson, S (2019) Sleep Comfortably, www.webmd.com

Godman, H (2012) Losing Weight And Belly Fat Improves Sleep, www.health.harvard.edu

Harvard Medical School (2013) Improving Sleep, Harvard Health Publishing

How Sleep Works (2019) 25 Weird Ways To Fall Asleep That Actually Work, www.howsleepworks.com

Kinman, T & Krucik, G (2015) Home Remedies For Restless Leg Syndrome, www.healthline.com

Koopman, D (2019) 10 Scientifically Proven Health Benefits Of Taking A Bath, www.lifehack.org

Kosecki, D (2018) REM, Light, Deep: How Much Of Each Stage Of Sleep Are You Getting? www.blog.fitbit.com

Mayo Clinic (2019) Sleep Apnea,
www.mayoclinic.org

National Sleep Foundation (2019) Aging and
Sleeping, www.sleepfoundation.org

Phillips, K (2014) How To Stop Snoring ASAP,
www.alaskasleep.com

Robinson, L. Segal, R. & Smith, M. (2019)
Sleeping Pills And Natural Sleep Aids,
www.helpguide.org

Sakugawa, Y (2015) 8 Weird Tips To Help You
Fall   Asleep,
www.thesecretyumiverse.wonderhowto.com

Semeco, A (2017) 20 Simple Tips That Help You
Fall Asleep Quickly, www.healthline.com

Sleep Advisor, (2019) 45 Sleep Mantras Better
Than Counting Sheep, www.sleepadvisor.org

Steber, C (2016) 11 Weird Tips For Falling Asleep
That Can Actually Work, www.bustle.com

Unknown (2018) Improving Your Deep Sleep
Naturally, www.hafco.co.uk

Unknown (2018) How Sleep Works (2018)
www.tuck.com

Unknown, (nd)19 Things To Try When You Can't
Sleep (Better Than Staring At A Clock),
www.synonymoussail.com

Zeratsky, K (2018) Is Too Little Sleep A Cause Of Weight Gain? www.mayoclinic.org

Zipkin, N (2017) 20 Weird Strategies To Help You Sleep, www.entrepreneur.com

Connect With The Author

www.debbiebrewer.co.uk

https://www.facebook.com/DebbieBrewerPoetry

www.instagram.com/poetrytreasures

www.twitter.com/poetrytreasure

www.ingramcontent.com/pod-product-compliance
Lightning Source LLC
Chambersburg PA
CBHW060505290526
45791CB00001B/276